Wall Pilates Workouts For Seniors

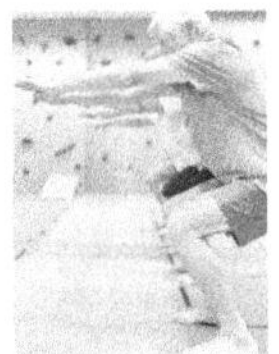

The Complete illustrated balance exercises to improve strength and flexibility for people over 60

Table of contents

Introduction

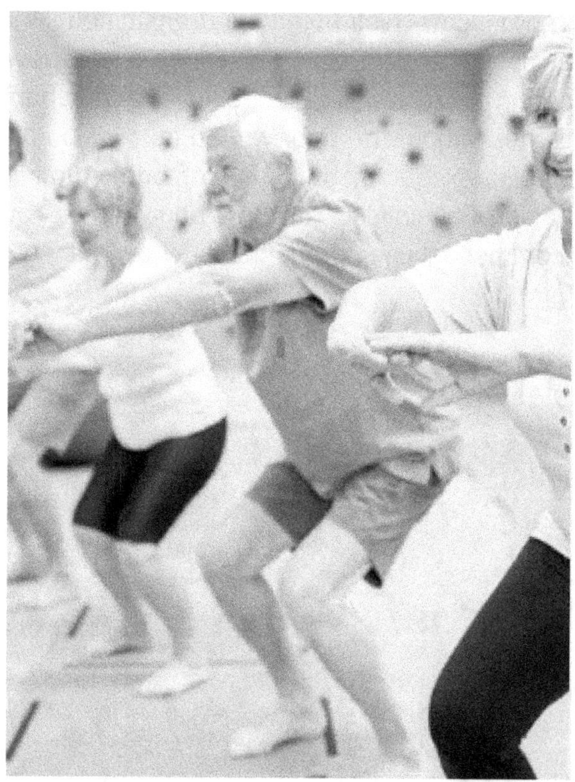

In a quaint town nestled between rolling hills and charming landscapes, lived a vibrant community of seniors who cherished their golden years. However, a common predicament began to unfold among them—stiffness, limited mobility, and a yearning for rejuvenation.

Meet Mrs. Thompson, a spirited resident whose zest for life was hindered by the challenges that often accompany aging. As her once agile limbs faced resistance, she found herself yearning for a solution to restore the vitality that once defined her daily pursuits.

Enter **Rena J. Deangelo**, a dedicated physiotherapist with a passion for holistic well-being. Recognizing the prevalent struggle among the seniors in her community, Dr. Turner embarked on a mission to unveil a transformative solution—Wall Pilates Workouts for Seniors.

The problem was clear—the community was yearning for a way to enhance flexibility, improve strength, and reignite their zest for life. **Rena J. Deangelo**, armed with her expertise, introduced Wall Pilates as the beacon of hope. This innovative approach, specifically tailored for seniors, utilized the support of walls to ensure safety while delivering effective exercises to address their unique needs.

In the heart of the community center, Mrs. Thompson and her peers gathered to experience the gentle yet powerful movements of Wall Pilates. The sessions were designed to alleviate joint stiffness, enhance balance, and promote overall well-being.

As the group embraced this rejuvenating journey, they discovered a newfound sense of strength and resilience.

The ultimate solution to their needs unfolded within the pages of "Wall Pilates Workouts For Seniors." **Rena J. Deangelo**, with her comprehensive guide, offered not just a set of exercises but a pathway to renewed vitality. The book became a trusted companion, providing step-by-step instructions, safety considerations, and a holistic approach to health.

As the community members dove into the Wall Pilates workouts, a remarkable transformation took place. Mrs. Thompson, once constrained by physical limitations, found herself reclaiming the joy of movement. The community echoed with laughter, resilience, and a shared sense of accomplishment.

The story of Mrs. Thompson and her fellow residents became a testament to the transformative power of Wall Pilates, proving that age is no barrier to embracing a vibrant and active lifestyle. **Rena J. Deangelo's** book became more than just a guide—it became a beacon of empowerment, helping seniors rediscover the joy of movement, one Wall Pilates workout at a time.

Chapter 1

Benefits for Seniors

Seniors can benefit greatly from wall Pilates, which enhances general wellbeing. In the context of the book "Wall Pilates Workouts for Seniors," the benefits section would go into further detail about the advantages that this particular type of exercise has for elderly citizens. This is a synopsis:

Better alignment of posture:

Seniors can maintain a more erect and balanced posture by placing emphasis on alignment and core engagement.
reduction of typical problems including back discomfort and tense muscles brought on by bad posture.
Enhanced Stability and Core Strength:

Exercises that target the core muscles increase stability and strength.

In addition to being essential for daily tasks, core strength can help seniors avoid falling, which is a typical concern.

Flexibility and Range of Motion of Joints:

Stretching gently against a wall enhances range of motion and joint flexibility.

especially advantageous for elderly people with stiffness or arthritis.

Minimal-Impact Environment:

Wall Pilates is a low-impact exercise regimen that relieves joint stress and lowers the chance of injury.

Ideal for people with different levels of fitness and those who have joint issues.

Tone and Endurance of Muscles:

Progressive training tones and builds muscle without overtaxing the body.

Increased total functional fitness and assistance for daily tasks are derived from improved muscle endurance.

Mind-Body Link:

A strong mind-body connection can be fostered through mindful exercise and breath awareness.

promotes mental health by encouraging elders to live in the present.

Reducing Stress:

Stress and anxiety can be decreased by incorporating breathing exercises and relaxation methods.

a comprehensive strategy for fitness that takes into account both the mental and physical components of wellbeing.

Participation in Society:

Group Wall Pilates courses can promote social interaction and a sense of community.

Positive view on life and general mental health depend on social involvement.

The book hopes to encourage seniors to embrace Wall Pilates as a worthwhile and pleasurable workout program that enhances their general health and energy by emphasizing these advantages.

Safety Considerations

Consultation with Medical Specialists:

Give advice on the kinds of medical experts to contact, such as doctors, PTs, or specialists, depending on the patient's specific needs.

Emphasize how important it is to talk about any recent surgeries, long-term illnesses, or other health issues that might affect their capacity to exercise.
Exercise Personalization:

Give examples of how to adjust exercises to suit different levels of physical ability and fitness.
Seniors should be encouraged to concentrate on form rather than intensity, and each exercise should provide visual signals or instructions for optimal posture.
Gradual Advancement:

Stress the idea of progressing gradually to prevent overdoing and lower the chance of harm.
Encourage a methodical approach to escalating the amount of challenge in the exercises, considering the comfort and confidence of the person.
Understanding Body Language:

Describe the common symptoms of overexertion, such as sudden discomfort, lightheadedness, or dyspnea.
Seniors should be encouraged to be proactive in addressing any issues regarding their physical well-being and to have open communication with their healthcare practitioners.
A suitable warm-up and cool-down

Offer a sequence of warm-up exercises designed to target the particular muscles used in Wall Pilates.

Stress the importance of a cool-down regimen for increasing flexibility and lowering post-workout muscular tightness.

Utilizing Appropriate Equipment:

Describe the different kinds of equipment used in wall Pilates and how to keep it safe and in good working order.

Provide substitutes for individuals who might not possess particular equipment, encouraging adaptability in exercise regimens.

Fall Safety:

Workout routines should include workouts that improve balance.

Stress how crucial it is to have a sturdy support—like a chair or wall—when performing balance-challenging exercises.

Nutrition and Hydration:

Emphasize how maintaining adequate fluids can reduce weariness and promote general wellness.

Give seniors fundamental dietary advice and encourage them to keep a balanced diet that complements their exercise regimen.

Emergency Planning and Medical Alerts:

Talk about the need of keeping medical records on hand, particularly for those who have long-term illnesses.

Describe emergency protocols and give advice on how to manage typical problems like lightheadedness or dyspnea during physical activity.

Frequent Check-Ins:

Stress the value of routine check-ins with medical specialists to track progress and modify the fitness regimen as needed.

To guarantee continued support and direction, seniors and their healthcare providers should communicate frequently.

The book intends to provide seniors the confidence to participate in Wall Pilates by thoroughly covering these safety concerns and equipping them with the knowledge and resources to put their health and safety first throughout their fitness journey.

Chapter 2

Getting Started

Essential Equipment

Yoga Mat:

For floor-based workouts, a cozy, non-slip yoga mat offers a stable platform.
During Pilates exercises, it provides additional padding for the knees, spine, and other sensitive areas.
Robust Wall Area:

When performing activities that require leaning, pressing, or holding the body against the wall, use a clear, stable wall area.
Make sure there are no obstructions and plenty of room to move around the wall.
Ball for exercise:

Exercise balls are useful for a range of wall-based stability and core-strengthening activities.
It introduces an element of instability by causing some actions to engage the deeper core muscles.
Bands of Resistance:

In order to build muscle strength and endurance, resistance bands offer a gentle approach to add resistance to a variety of workouts.
They are adaptable and work well against walls in exercises for the upper and lower bodies.
Fit Ring (Magic Circle) Pilates:

A flexible circle called a Pilates ring can increase the resistance and intensity of some workouts.
It's especially helpful for improving total muscle engagement and targeting the inner and outer thighs.
Athletic Shoes That Are Comfy:

Seniors who perform dynamic and standing exercises should wear supportive and comfortable sporting shoes to ensure stability.
A strong arch supporter in a shoe can enhance overall safety.
Stability bar or chair:

For balance-focused activities, it can be helpful to have a wall-mounted stability bar or a stable chair nearby to offer additional support.

It's especially helpful for people who are new to Pilates or seniors who might require extra help.

Bottle of water:

During any exercise, it's critical to stay hydrated. Urge elderly people to always have a bottle of water handy so they may take a sip as needed.

Staying well hydrated promotes general wellbeing and reduces weariness.

Easy-to-wear attire:

Seniors should dress in comfortable, breathable attire that doesn't restrict their range of motion.

Wearing comfortable clothing guarantees a successful and joyful workout.

Stopwatch or timer:

A timer or stopwatch can help elders pace themselves and monitor their progress during scheduled exercises or intervals.

It gives the exercise regimen structure and permits appropriate rest periods.

Setting Up Your Workout Space

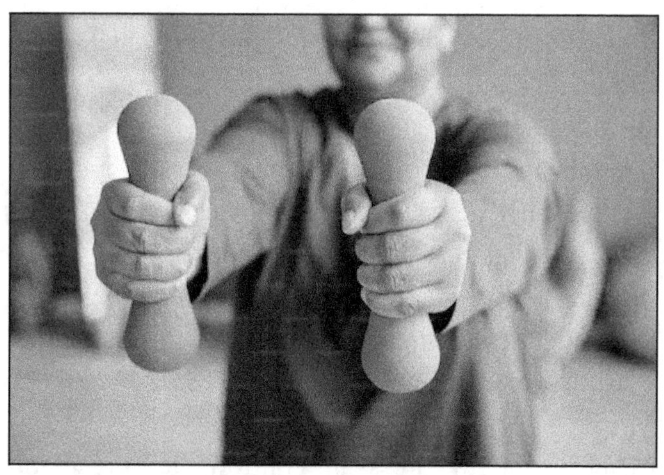

Choosing the Correct Room:

Select a room that has adequate natural light, ventilation, and room to move around.
Make sure there are no trip hazards and that the floor is level.
Making Room:

Clear the area of any furniture, objects, or obstructions that might impede your movements.
Make a space free of clutter to guarantee everyone's safety when exercising.
Selecting an Appropriate Wall:

Select a wall with sufficient room for pressing and leaning exercises that is clear of clutter.

Make sure there are no protruding objects and that the wall is stable.

Where to Put a Yoga Mat:

Your yoga mat should be set up in the middle of the exercise area.

For floor workouts, the mat offers a cozy surface and increases traction to stop slipping.

Equipment Positioning for Exercise:

Place Pilates rings, resistance bands, exercise balls, and other equipment in convenient locations.

Arrange the equipment so that there are as little disruptions as possible when working out.

Getting Appropriate Lighting

Make sure there is enough light so you can see your body alignment properly and securely do the exercises.

While natural light is ideal, bright artificial lighting can be used in its place.

Temperature regulation and ventilation:

To avoid pain or overheating, keep the environment at a suitable temperature.

Make sure there is enough ventilation to maintain clean air when working out.

Having a Chair or Stability Bar Close by:

Put a wall-mounted stability bar or a sturdy chair within easy reach.
This offers extra aid when performing balance-focused workouts, particularly for elderly people who might require it.
Setting Up the Towel and Water:

Keep a little towel and a water bottle close by.
It's important to stay hydrated, and you can use a towel to wipe away perspiration while working out.
Establishing a Positive Environment

Think about selecting a workout time that corresponds with the person's peak energy levels or turning on soothing music.
Promote the development of a joyful and upbeat workout environment.
Customizing the Area:

To make the area welcoming, add unique touches like inspirational sayings, beloved colors, or upbeat décor.
An room dedicated to your workout can improve the whole experience.

Warm-Up Exercises

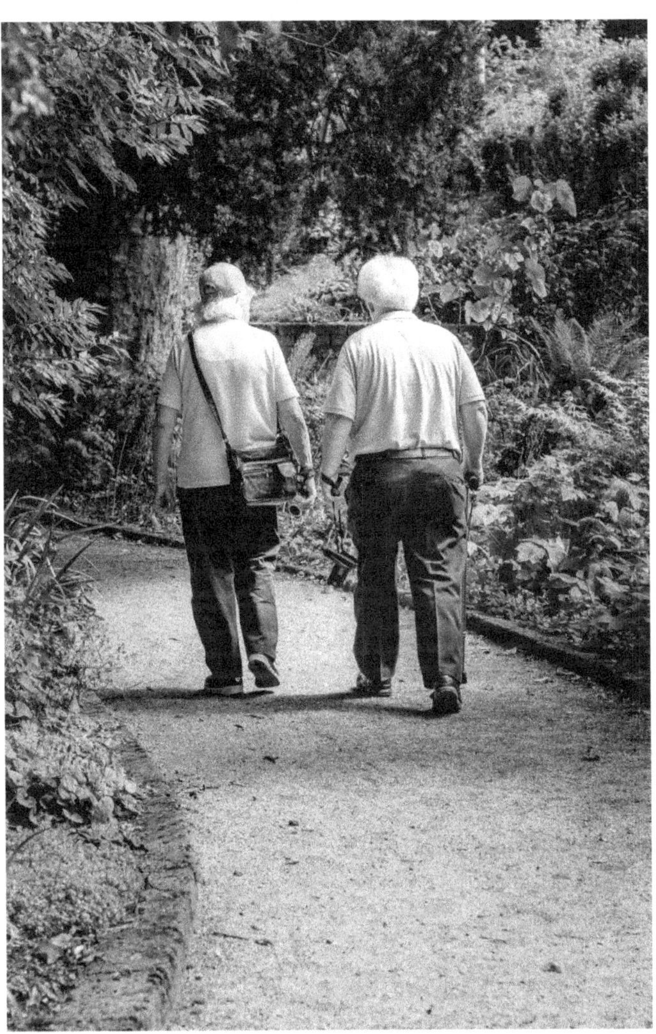

Rolls of the neck:

Move the neck in a gentle clockwise and counterclockwise circular motion.
This enhances flexibility and relieves tension in the neck.
Rolls of the shoulders:

Raise shoulders to ear level, then gently roll them back and forth in a circle.
relaxes the upper back and shoulders.
Arm Rotations:

Move your arms in a deliberate, forward and backward motion.
This enhances range of motion and helps warm up the shoulder joints.
Torso Rotations:

Place your feet hip-width apart and rotate your upper body in a circular motion.
activates the core and gets the spine ready for motion.
Circles in the hips:

Place your hands on your hips and make a circular motion with your hips.
a mild method for increasing hip joint warmth and range of motion.
Knee Extensions:

While standing, raise each knee alternately toward the chest.
activates the hip flexors and warms the lower body.
Ankle Rings:

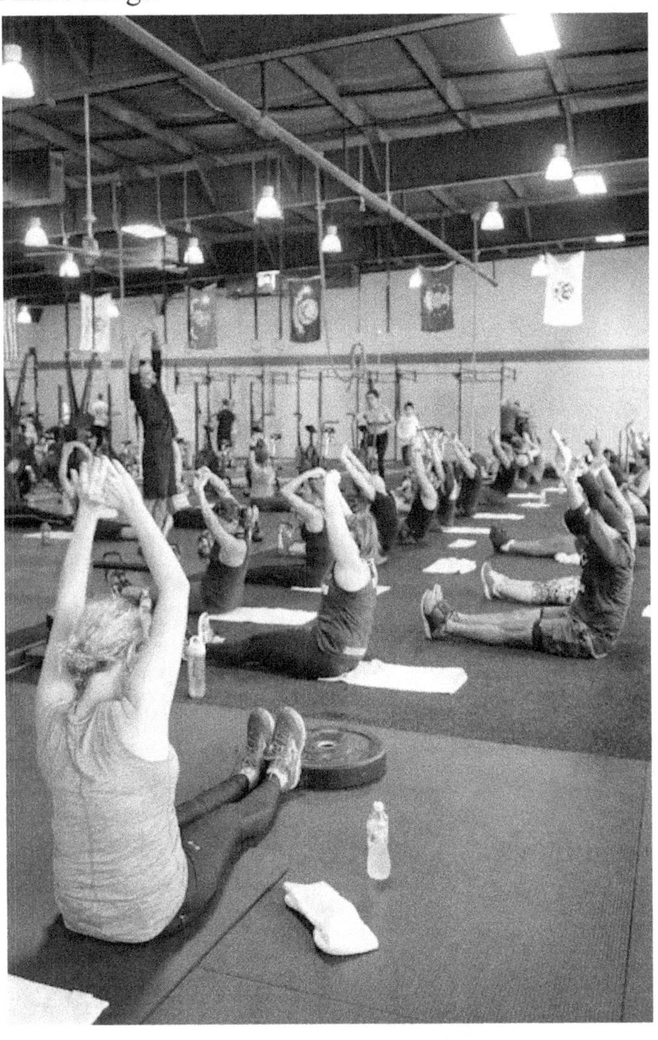

Rotate the ankle in both clockwise and counterclockwise directions while elevating one foot.
To warm up the ankles, repeat with the other foot.
March at the Location:

March by raising your knees and softly pumping your arms.
raises heart rate and promotes bodily warmth.
Heel Lifts:

Place your heels up off the ground and then place them back down while keeping your feet hip-width apart.
heats the lower limbs and strengthens the calf muscles.
Push-ups against the wall:

With your back to the wall, position your hands shoulder-height on the wall.
To warm up the arms and chest, perform a series of controlled push-ups against the wall.
Inhaling deeply:

Throughout the warm-up, use deep, rhythmic breathing to oxygenate the body and soothe the mind.

Chapter 3

Foundation Exercises

Wall Squats

Tools Required:

Wall   Yoga   Mat: Requirements   and recommendations:

Initial Position:

Make sure your feet are hip-width apart while you stand with your back to a wall.
One can place their feet 12 to 18 inches away from the wall.

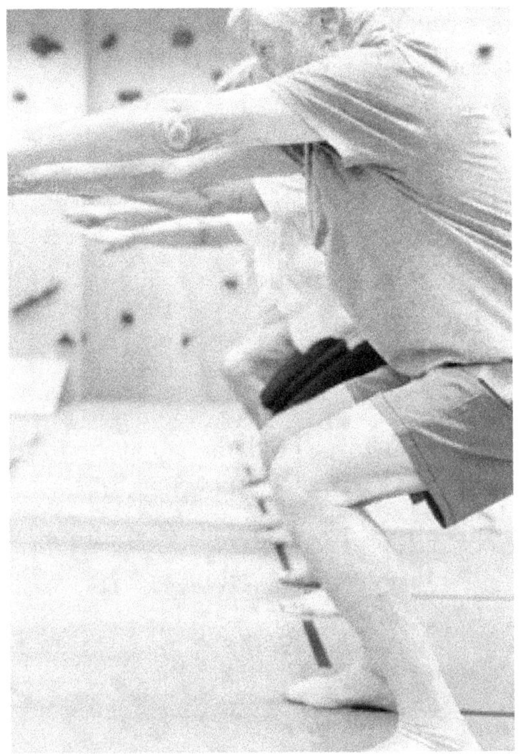

Work Your Core Muscles:

To activate your core, bring your navel in close to your spine.
Maintain your back against the wall while letting your shoulders drop.
Scooping Down:

As you slowly descend the wall, bend your knees and bring your body down to sit.

Make sure your knees stay just above your ankles and do not extend past your toes.
Position of Squat:

As low as your comfort will allow, lower your body until your thighs are parallel to the floor.
Try to squat in a position that feels comfortable, avoiding any knee pain.
Take a Hold and Inhale:

With proper posture, hold the squat position for a few breaths.
Make an effort to maintain a uniform weight distribution through your feet.
Getting Up:

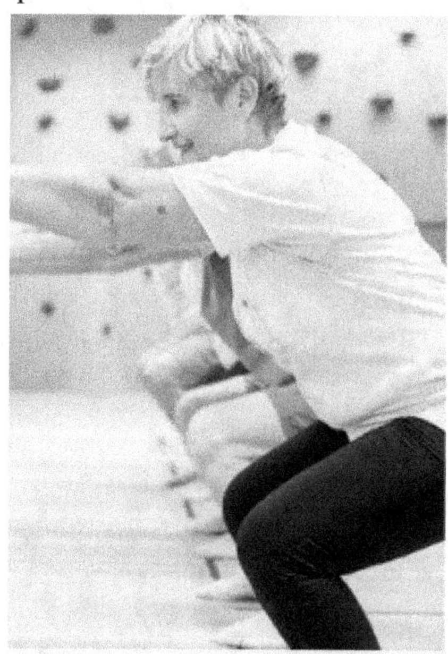

To slowly stand back up, put pressure on your heels and tighten your thigh muscles.

Throughout the exercise, keep your back against the wall.

Again:

Do ten to fifteen repetitions, or however many are comfortable for you.

The number of repetitions can be gradually increased as you get more accustomed to the workout.

Advice:

Reduce the depth of the squat or use a smaller range of motion if you are experiencing knee pain.

To avoid putting undue strain on your joints, make sure your knees remain in line with your toes.

Pay close attention to deliberate motions and emphasize using your glute and thigh muscles.

Advantages:

hamstrings, glutes, and quadriceps are strengthened.

increases the endurance of the lower body.

improves equilibrium and steadiness.

offers a low-impact way to strengthen your lower body.

Wall Bridges

Tools Required:

Wall Yoga Mat: Requirements and recommendations:

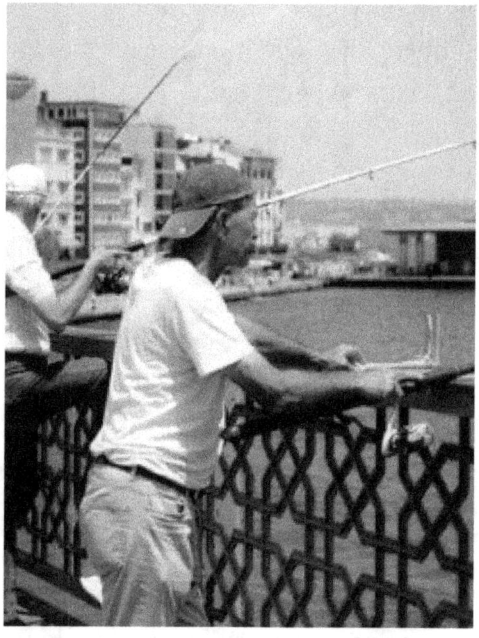

Initial Position:

Lay flat on your back with your feet hip-width apart and your knees bent.
With your palms facing down, place your arms by your sides.
Modify Wall Proximity:

Move your heels closer to the wall until they are between six and twelve inches from it.
Make sure your lower back, in particular, is resting comfortably on the floor.
Work Your Core Muscles:

To activate your core muscles, pull your navel forward toward your spine.
Maintain a relaxed neck and softly press your shoulders onto the ground.
Raise Your Hips Up to the Ceiling:

Elevate your hips toward the ceiling by applying pressure with your heels.
At the peak of the exercise, your body should be in a straight line from your shoulders to your knees.
Maintain the Bridge Position:

For a short while, hold the bridge posture while concentrating on keeping your body straight and contracting your glutes.
Make sure your feet and shoulders receive the same amount of weight.
Scooping Down:

With control, slowly return your hips to their initial position.

Steer clear of abrupt dips and instead use slow, fluid movements.
Again:

Do ten to fifteen repetitions, or however many are comfortable for you.
Once you get more comfortable with the activity, you can progressively up the number of reps.
Advice:

Aim for a straight line from your shoulders to your knees when performing the bridge to avoid overly arching your lower back.

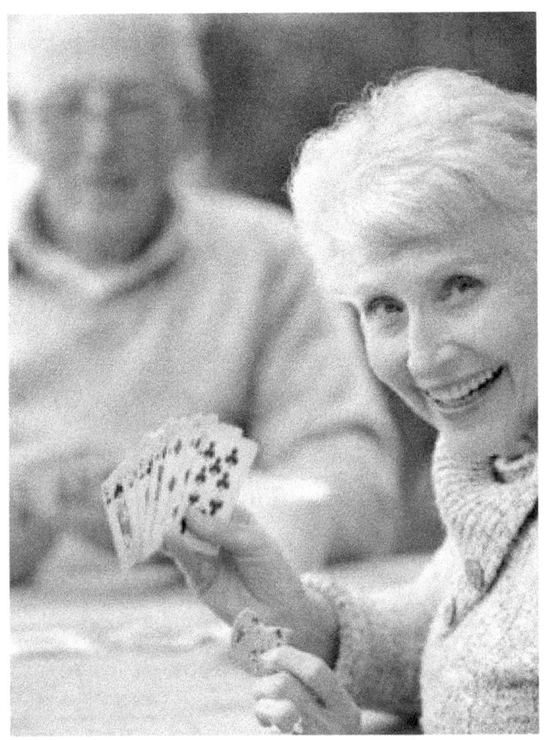

Instead of depending exclusively on your lower back to raise your hips, concentrate on engaging your hamstrings and glutes.
Advantages:

strengthens the lower back, hamstrings, and glutes.
enhances pelvic alignment and central stability.
increases hip articulation.
offers a mild method of activating the posterior chain without straining the spine.

Leg Lifts with Wall Support

Tools Required:

Wall Yoga Mat: Requirements and recommendations:

Initial Position:

Stretch your legs out along the wall while lying on your back.
With your palms facing down, place your hands by your sides.
Work Your Core Muscles:

To activate your core, bring your navel in close to your spine.
Make sure your lower back is softly pressed into the ground.
Leg raises:

Straightening both legs, raise them toward the ceiling.
Put your hands on the ground or firmly press them up against the wall to get support from it.
Managed Motion:

Controlfully lower your legs back down toward the wall.

Try to keep your movement slow and deliberate in order to properly use your muscles.
Steer clear of lower back arching:

Make sure your lower back touches the floor at all times during the exercise.
Minimize your range of motion or slightly bend your knees if you feel your lower back elevating.
Again:

Do ten to fifteen repetitions, or however many are comfortable for you.
Pay more attention to the type of movement than the amount.
Advice:

As your strength increases, start with a smaller range of motion and progressively expand it.
Maintain a relaxed neck and a pressed-in posture with your shoulders.
Throughout the workout, take steady breaths, exhaling as you raise your legs and inhaling as you lower them.
Advantages:

makes the muscles in the lower abdomen stronger.
focuses on the thighs and hip flexors.
increases core stability all around.

offers a supporting and controlled substitute for conventional leg raises.

Seniors should adjust the movement to their comfort level and pay attention to how their body responds, just like with any other workout. Before adding new activities to their program, it's advisable to speak with a healthcare provider if there are any concerns or pre-existing health conditions.

Chapter 4

Core Strengthening

Wall Planks

Tools Required:

Wall Yoga Mat: Requirements and recommendations:

Initial Position:

Put your hands shoulder-height on the wall while facing the wall.

Reposition your feet so that your torso is in a straight line from your head to your heels.
Placement of the Hand:

Make sure your hands are parallel to your shoulders and spaced shoulder-width apart.
Spread your digits to enhance steadiness.
Work Your Core Muscles:

To activate your core, bring your navel in close to your spine.
From your head to your heels, keep your body in a straight line; don't droop or arch.
Maintain the Plank Position:

For 20 to 30 seconds, or for as long as it is comfortable, maintain the plank posture.
Pay attention to keeping your shoulders squarely above your wrists and maintaining a neutral spine.
Inhaling:

Throughout the plank, breathe steadily and do not hold your breath.
Breathe in from your nose, out through your mouth.
Gradual Advancement:

As you get more accustomed to the exercise, try to extend the plank's duration.

For an extra challenge while keeping your balance, try lifting one foot off the ground.
Scooping Down:

To get out of the plank posture, slowly return your feet to the wall.
If necessary, give your wrists a shake.
Advice:

To avoid putting too much strain on the lower back, concentrate on using your core muscles.
To prevent locking your elbows, maintain a small bend in them.
To keep your alignment correct, make sure your neck is in a neutral position and your eyes are on the floor.
Advantages:

bolsters the arms, shoulders, and core.
enhances balance and stability all around.
uses a variety of muscular areas without straining the wrists.
provides a safe and regulated alternative to conventional planks.
Seniors should listen to their body, begin with a time that seems comfortable, and go at their own pace when exercising, just like with any other kind of exercise. Before adding new activities to their program, it's advisable to speak with a healthcare

provider if there are any concerns or pre-existing health conditions.

Modified Side Planks

Tools Required:

Wall Yoga Mat: Requirements and recommendations:

Initial Position:

With your forearm lying on the floor and your elbow precisely beneath your shoulder, lie on your side.
Place your feet behind you, stack your legs on top of one another, and bend your knees.
Placement of the Hand:

For support, rest your free hand on the ground in front of you.
Make sure your hand is positioned just a little bit broader than your shoulder.
Work Your Core Muscles:

To activate your core, bring your navel in close to your spine.
Raise your hips off the ground so that your head and knees are in a straight line.
Grip the Adapted Side Plank:

Hold this posture for 15 to 30 seconds, or for whatever long it is comfortable for you.
Make an effort to maintain a straight body and refrain from sagging or twisting.
Inhaling:

Throughout the plank, breathe steadily and do not hold your breath.
Breathe in from your nose, out through your mouth.
Gradual Advancement:

As you get more accustomed to the exercise, try to extend the plank's duration.
To add even more challenge without compromising balance, try elevating your upper leg.
Scooping Down:

To get out of the modified side plank, gently lower your hips back to the floor.
Repeat the exercise by switching to the opposite side.
Advice:

Maintain a neutral neck posture while focusing directly ahead.

To raise your hips, concentrate on using the muscles on the side of your body.

Make sure your hand is in the best place to provide stability.

Advantages:

obliques, or side abdominal muscles, are strengthened.

increases equilibrium and core stability.

Work the arm and shoulder muscles gently.

provides a senior-friendly version that has been modified.

Seniors should listen to their body, begin with a duration that is comfortable, and increase at their own speed when exercising, just like with any other physical activity. Before adding new activities to their program, it's advisable to speak with a healthcare provider if there are any concerns or pre-existing health conditions.

Abdominal Exercises Against the Wall

Tools Required:

Yoga mat on the wall (optional)
Wall Crunches: How to Do It:

Lay flat on your back with your legs bent and your feet flat against the wall.

Either cross your hands over your chest or place them behind your head.

Bring your chest towards your knees by using your core to raise your head, shoulders, and chest off the mat.

As you crunch up, release your breath and inhale as you descend again.

Do this 12–15 times over.

2. Instructions for Leg Raises Against the Wall:

Lay flat on your back with your legs straight up against the wall and your buttocks near to the wall.

For support, place your hands beneath your hips or at your sides.

Keep your legs from touching as you sag toward the floor.

As you raise your legs back to the beginning position, release the breath.

Do this 12–15 times over.

3. Knee Tuck Wall Plank Instructions:

With your hands on the floor immediately beneath your shoulders and your feet pressed against the wall, begin in the plank position.

Bring your right knee up to your chest while using your core.

Repeat with the left knee after putting the right foot back against the wall.

Do 12–15 repetitions of alternate knee tucks on each leg.

Advice for Doing Abdominal Workouts Up against the Wall:

Keep Your Alignment Correct:

To prevent stressing the lower back, keep your back flat against the mat or floor.

Make sure the position of your spine, head, and neck is neutral.

Managed Motions:

Make sure to contract the abdominal muscles during each regulated movement.

Do not raise or lower your upper or lower body with momentum.

Inhaling:

Breathe in sync with every movement. When lifting the head or legs, for example, you should exhale during the exertion phase and inhale during the relaxation period.

Modify Intensity:

Depending on your level of fitness, adjust the number of repetitions or the range of motion.
If a workout seems too hard, scale it down until you gain strength and self-assurance.
Wall Assist:

When you need support and stability, especially if you're new to abdominal workouts or are worried about your balance, use the wall.
These wall-mounted abdominal workouts work a variety of core muscles, enhancing strength and stability. Seniors should constantly pay attention to their bodies, adjust activities as necessary, and seek medical advice if they have any underlying medical illnesses or concerns.

Chapter 5

Balance and Stability

Wall Lunges

Tools Required:

Yoga mat on the wall (optional)
Wall Lunges: How to Do It:

Initial Position:

Place your feet about hip-width apart and face the wall.
For support, place your hands at shoulder height on the wall.
Take a Backseat:

With your right foot, walk back while keeping your distance from the wall.
When you lunge, make sure your feet are hip-width apart.
Plunge Motion:

Lower your body toward the floor by bending both of your knees.

Maintain a straight front knee over your ankle and a back knee that is pointed down toward the ground.

Keep Your Posture Straight:

Maintain an erect posture and elevate your chest.

For stability, contract your core muscles.

Return to Starting Position by Pushing:

To get back to where you were, push through the front foot's heel.

Assure deliberate and fluid motions.

Different Legs:

Using the opposing leg, perform the lunge motion again.

For 12–15 reps on each leg, keep switching up your legs.

A Few Wall Lunge Tips:

Appropriate Alignment

Keep your body in good alignment by positioning your back knee to point toward the floor and your front knee just above your ankle.

Remain upright with your torso and avoid bending too much forward.

Managed Motions:

Avoid making sudden or jerky movements when performing the lunges. Instead, move carefully.

During the workout, concentrate on using your leg muscles.

Inhaling:

Sync your breathing with the motions. Breathe in as you descend into the lunge and out as you ascend again.

Wall Assist:

As needed, use the wall as support. Placing your hands on the wall can help add support if you're having trouble staying balanced.

Flexibility of Movement:

As you get more accustomed to the exercise, progressively increase the range of motion from where you started.

Should you feel any pain, shallow down the lunge.

Prioritizing safety

Before doing wall lunges, see a healthcare provider if you have any current knee or joint problems.

If you feel pain or discomfort throughout the activity, pay attention to your body and stop.

Wall lunges are a low-impact lower body strengthening exercise that may be modified to accommodate different levels of fitness. Seniors should adjust the movement to their comfort level and ability, like with any exercise, to provide a safe and efficient workout.

Single Leg Stands

Particularly for seniors, single-leg stands are great workouts for increasing leg strength, stability, and balance. To increase safety, these workouts can be modified to include wall support. Here's how to do single-leg stands against the wall step-by-step:

Tools Required:

Yoga mat on the wall (optional)
Directions for Single-Leg Stands Against the Wall:

Initial Position:

Place your feet hip-width apart and lean back against the wall.
For support, place your hands at shoulder height on the wall.
Adjust Weight to Just One Leg:

Elevate your left foot a few inches off the ground and shift your weight onto your right leg.

On your right leg, find a secure and comfortable position.

Work Your Core Muscles:

To keep your posture stable and erect, contract your core muscles.

Stay away from leaning on the wall; it is just meant to provide minimal support when needed.

Maintain the Position:

For 15 to 30 seconds, or for as long as it feels comfortable, maintain the single-leg position.

To aid with balance, fix your attention on something in front of you or on the wall.

Turn to Your Other Leg:

As you move your weight to your left leg, lower your left foot to the floor.

Find a secure position by lifting your right foot a few inches off the ground.

Hold and carry out again:

For 15 to 30 seconds, maintain the single-leg position on your left leg.

For three to five repetitions on each leg, keep switching between the legs.

Advice for Standing on One Leg Against a Wall:
Wall Assist:

When you need light support, use the wall. Rather than carrying the entire weight, its purpose is to offer stability.
Keep Your Alignment Correct:

Make sure your knee is in line with your toes and maintain a tiny bend in your standing leg.
Ensure that your shoulders are above your hips and that you are erect.
Work Your Core Muscles:

Bring your navel in close to your spine to engage your core muscles.
During the workout, this enhances balance and stability.
Consistent Breathing:

Breathe continuously while performing the activity.
Breathe in and out slowly and deliberately.
Pay Attention to Balance:

To aid in balancing, focus on locating a focal point.
To make your balance even more difficult, consider closing your eyes for a little while, if it feels comfortable.
Gradual Advancement:

As your balance gets better, extend each single-leg stand.
Reduce your rely on the wall for support bit by bit.
Prioritizing safety

Use a stable surface or the assistance of someone close if you struggle with balance or other concerns. Seniors can improve their balance and leg strength in a safe and efficient manner by using single-leg stands against walls. As usual, it's crucial to carry out workouts within a comfortable range and speak with a medical expert if there are any underlying health issues.

Toe Taps and Heel Raises

A senior-friendly exercise program can benefit from the incorporation of basic yet efficient movements like toe taps and heel lifts to enhance ankle strength, balance, and overall lower body stability. These exercises are especially helpful for seniors who want to improve their mobility and lower their chance of falling. This is a tutorial on how to raise your heel and do toe taps:

Tools Required:

Support from a sturdy chair or wall Toe Taps:
Directions:

Initial Position:

With your feet hip-width apart, take an upright stance and face a sturdy chair or wall for support.
Make sure each of your feet are bearing the same amount of weight.
Point your toes forward:

Raise your right foot a little and tap the floor with your toes.
Place your right foot back where it was initially.
Different Legs:

Tap your toes forward while slightly elevating your left foot.
Continue doing ten to fifteen reps on each leg, switching between your right and left toes.
Keep Your Posture Straight:

Throughout the exercise, maintain your upper body straight, shoulders relaxed, and core engaged.
Heel Raises: Guideline:

Initial Position:

With your feet hip-width apart, take an upright stance and face a sturdy chair or wall for support.
Make sure each of your feet are bearing the same amount of weight.
Take Your Shoes Off the Ground:

Raise yourself onto the balls of your feet by gradually lifting both heels off the ground.
Hold the posture up for a brief period of time.
Bring Your Heels Down:

Releasing your heels to the floor with gentleness while keeping your balance.
Make sure your heels come into controlled contact with the floor.
Again:

Heel lifts should be done ten to fifteen times; as your strength increases, progressively increase the amount of reps.
Keep Your Posture Straight:

Throughout the exercise, maintain your upper body straight, shoulders relaxed, and core engaged.
Advice on Heel Raises and Toe Taps:
Employ Assistance:

If you're new to these exercises or have trouble with your balance, specifically, hold onto a strong chair or use a wall as support.
Managed Motions:

To optimize muscle engagement and improve balance, execute the actions slowly and deliberately.
Inhaling:

Breathe in rhythm with the movements. Breathe in during the preparatory phase and out during the effort period.
Gradual Advancement:

As your strength and balance improve, start with a limited range of motion and progressively increase it.
Prioritizing safety

If you have any health issues or balance problems already, try these exercises on a stable surface or with a support person nearby.
A senior-friendly workout regimen would benefit greatly from the addition of toe taps and heel lifts, which are low-impact yet very efficient ways to improve ankle strength and overall lower body stability. Before beginning a new workout regimen, always put safety first and see a medical expert if you have any health-related concerns.

Chapter 6

Flexibility and Range of Motion

Wall Stretching Routine

A senior-friendly exercise program can benefit greatly from a wall stretching practice since it increases range of motion, flexibility, and relaxation. These wall stretches are geared toward senior citizens. It's wise to speak with a healthcare provider before beginning any new fitness regimen, particularly if there are any current health issues. Make sure you complete these stretches in a range of motion that is pain-free, and cease the stretch immediately if you experience any discomfort.

Tools Required:

Wall 1. Wall Chest Stretch: Assume a wall-facing position.

Press your forearm and right hand up against the wall.

Feel a stretch across your chest and in front of your shoulder as you slowly rotate your body to the left.

After 15 to 30 seconds of holding, switch sides.

2. Wall Shoulder Stretch: Face the wall obliquely.

Place the palm of your right arm against the wall and extend it to shoulder height.

As you turn your body away from the wall, your shoulders should feel stretched.

After 15 to 30 seconds of holding, switch sides.

3. Wall Calf Stretch: Place your hands shoulder-height on the wall while facing the wall.

Maintaining a straight right foot, take a step back.

Feel for a stretch in your right calf as you press your right heel onto the floor.

After 15 to 30 seconds of holding, switch sides.

4. Wall Hip Flexor Stretch: Stand facing the wall with your hands resting on it for stability.

Retrace your right foot while bending your knee a little.

Press your hips forward softly while maintaining a modest bend in your left knee.

Your right hip's front feels stretched out.

After 15 to 30 seconds of holding, switch sides.

5. Wall Hamstring Stretch: Lean your left side against the wall while seated on the floor.

Lean your left leg outward against the wall.

Reach for your toes with your hips like a hinge.

Your left leg's back should feel stretched.

After 15 to 30 seconds of holding, switch sides.

6. Wall Lower Back Stretch: Assume a prone position, bringing your buttocks near the wall.

Raise your legs up against the wall.

Let your arms hang loose at your sides.

You should feel a slight stretch in your hamstrings and lower back.

Breathe deeply while holding for one to two minutes.

7. Wall Ankle Stretch: Sit with your legs out in front of the wall.

Place the top of your flexed right foot against the wall.

Point your toes in the direction of the wall.

Your right ankle's back should feel stretched.

After 15 to 30 seconds of holding, switch sides.

Advice for Stretching Walls:

Reach Your Comfort Zone:

Only extend until you feel tension, not pain.

Reduce the intensity of the stretch if it hurts.

Grasp Every Stretch:

To give the muscles time to relax and lengthen, hold each stretch for at least 15 to 30 seconds.

Regular Breathing

Take regular, deep breaths while performing each stretch.
Breathe in from your nose, out through your mouth.
Flowing Changes:

Smoothly and slowly enter and exit each stretch.
Adjust as Necessary:

If you have trouble moving about, adjust the stretches or use extra props to help you.
Be Aware:

Observe your body's reaction to each stretch and note how it feels.
Adapt as necessary to your feelings.
Recall that the purpose of stretching is to preserve joint mobility and improve flexibility. Regularly perform these stretches to reap the benefits of heightened flexibility and less stress in your muscles.

Neck and Shoulder Stretches

Stretches for the neck and shoulders are crucial for reducing stress, increasing range of motion, and encouraging relaxation. You can include this series of stretches into your regular routine to help relieve the typical discomfort brought on by stress in your shoulders and neck. Make sure to stretch within your pain-free range of motion and with gentle movements. Before beginning a new stretching regimen, it is essential to speak with a healthcare provider if you currently have any neck or shoulder problems.

1. Neck Tilt Stretch: Maintain a straight back when sitting or standing.
Bring your right ear to your right shoulder by slowly tilting your head to the right.
Feel a stretch along the left side of your neck while you hold for 15 to 30 seconds.
Go back to the center and do the opposite side.
2. Neck Rotation Stretch: Maintain a straight back while sitting or standing.
Take a look behind your shoulder and turn your head to the right.
Hold for 15 to 30 seconds, allowing your neck to gently expand.
Go back to the center and do the opposite side.
3. Neck Flexor Stretch: Maintain a straight back while sitting or standing.
Feel the back of your neck stretch as you slowly bring your chin up to your chest.
Hold for a duration of 15-30 seconds.

Return your head to the beginning position with gentle lift.

4. Shoulder Roll: Take a seat or stand with a relaxed posture.

Raise your shoulders to your ears and shrug.

Make a circle with your shoulders as you roll them back.

For ten to fifteen seconds, repeat.

Turn around and extend your shoulders forward.

5. Shoulder Stretch: Raise your right arm to shoulder height across your chest.

Press your right arm gently toward your chest with your left hand.

Hold for 15 to 30 seconds until your right shoulder starts to extend.

Continue on the opposite side.

6. Upper Trapezius Stretch: Maintain a straight back whether sitting or standing.

Bring your right ear closer to your right shoulder by tilting your head to the right.

Press gently with your right hand on the left side of your head.

Feel the left upper trapezius stretch as you hold for 15 to 30 seconds.

Continue on the opposite side.

7. Behind-the-Back Shoulder Stretch: With your palm facing outward, reach your right hand down your back.

Raise and place your left hand behind your back, palm inside out.
Put your hands together if you can.
Hold for 15 to 30 seconds while noticing your shoulders getting stretched.
Repeat with the other hand on top after releasing.
Advice on Shoulder and Neck Stretches:
Mild Motions:

To prevent tension, move slowly and gently through each stretch.
Inhaling:

Take regular, deep breaths while performing each stretch.
Breathe in from your nose, out through your mouth.
Comfortable Scope:

Only extend until you feel tension, not pain.
Reduce the intensity of the stretch if it hurts.
Continuity:

Incorporate these stretches into your everyday regimen to preserve suppleness and alleviate stress.
Adjust as Necessary:

Adapt the stretches to your level of comfort and any physical restrictions.
Remain Aware:

Take note of your body's needs and modify the stretches accordingly.

Speak with a healthcare provider if you have any concerns.

Regularly incorporate these stretches for the neck and shoulders into your regimen to help release stress and enhance your general flexibility. It is imperative that you consult a healthcare provider for an appropriate assessment and direction if you are experiencing ongoing pain or discomfort.

Seated Wall Stretches

Stretching can be easily incorporated into your routine with seated wall stretches, especially for those who are elderly or have restricted mobility. Stretching like this is done while seated, with the assistance of a wall. Make sure to take your time and carefully stretch each area, paying attention to your breathing and just go as far as possible without experiencing any pain. Before beginning a new stretching regimen, it is advisable to speak with a healthcare provider if you have any current health issues.

1. Seated Neck Stretch: Sit with your legs straight out in front of you and your back against a wall.

Bring your right ear to your right shoulder by slowly tilting your head to the right.

Feel a stretch along the left side of your neck while you hold for 15 to 30 seconds.

Go back to the center and do the opposite side.

2. Seated Shoulder Stretch: Lean your legs straight out in front of you while sitting with your back to a wall.

Fold your right arm over your torso.

Press your right arm gently toward your chest with your left hand.

Hold for 15 to 30 seconds until your right shoulder starts to extend.

Proceed with the left arm in the same manner.

3. Seated Forward Bend: Take a seat with your legs straight out in front of you and your back against the wall.

Lean forward and hinge at the hips to extend your reach to your toes.

Feel a stretch down your hamstrings and lower back as you hold for 15 to 30 seconds.

Return to your seat slowly.

4. Seated Hip Opener: Lean your legs straight out in front of you while sitting with your back to the wall.

Bring your right foot's sole up on your inner left thigh while bending your right knee.

Hold for 15 to 30 seconds, or until your right hip starts to stretch.

Repeat on the other side after switching your legs.

5. Seated Spinal Twist: Sit with your legs straight out in front of you and your back against the wall.

With your right foot on the outside of your left knee, bend your right knee.

With your left elbow on the outside of your right knee, make a right twist.

Once you feel a stretch in your spine, hold for 15 to 30 seconds.

Continue on the opposite side.

6. Seated Inner Thigh Stretch: Sit with your legs apart and your back against the wall.

Keeping your knees bent, slide your feet outward.

Hold for 15 to 30 seconds, allowing your inner thighs to stretch.

Return your knees to your sides slowly.

Some Advice on Sitting Wall Stretches:

Utilize the Wall as Support:

When performing seated stretches, the wall can offer support and stability.

Inhaling:

Take regular, deep breaths while performing each stretch.

Breathe in from your nose, out through your mouth.

Mild Motions:

To prevent tension, move slowly and gently through each stretch.
Comfortable Scope:

Only extend until you feel tension, not pain.
Reduce the intensity of the stretch if it hurts.
Continuity:

Incorporate these stretches into your everyday regimen to preserve suppleness and alleviate stress.
Adjust as Necessary:

Adapt the stretches to your level of comfort and any physical restrictions.
Remain Aware:

Take note of your body's needs and modify the stretches accordingly.
Speak with a healthcare provider if you have any concerns.
You can increase overall mobility, decrease stress, and increase flexibility by including these seated wall stretches into your everyday practice. Always pay attention to your body's needs and modify the stretches to fit your comfort level. Consult a healthcare provider if you are experiencing ongoing discomfort or if you have any concerns.

Chapter 7

Cool Down and Relaxation

Gentle Wall-Based Stretches

For those who prefer or need extra assistance during their stretching exercise, gentle wall-based stretches can be especially helpful. These stretches make use of a wall's support and are meant to be easy on the body. As usual, it's important to stretch within your range of motion without experiencing pain. Additionally, before beginning a new stretching regimen, seek medical advice if you have any pre-existing health issues.

1. Wall Chest Opener: Place your feet hip-width apart and face a wall.
Put your hands shoulder-height against the wall.
Feel a stretch across your chest by bending forward gently while maintaining a straight arm position.
Breathe deeply while holding for 15 to 30 seconds.
Return to your standing position gradually.
2. Wall Arm Stretch: Face the wall with your side facing you while you stand or sit.

Stretch out your right arm and rest the palm shoulder-height on the wall.

You should feel a stretch over your arm and shoulder as you turn your body away from the wall.

After 15 to 30 seconds of holding, switch sides.

3. Wall-attached Forward Fold: Put your hands at chest height on the wall while facing it.

Take a step back, bend at the hips, and lower your body to the floor.

Feel a slight stretch in your lower back and hamstrings while maintaining a straight back.

After holding for 15 to 30 seconds, carefully stand back up.

4. Wall Seated Forward Bend: Take a seat with your legs straight out in front of you and your back against the wall.

Move your body closer to the wall so that your back rests against it and your legs are extended upward.

You should feel a slight stretch in your lower back and hamstrings.

Breathe deeply while holding for one to two minutes.

5. Wall Calf Stretch: Put your hands against the wall while you stand facing it.

Retrace your steps with your right foot straight and heel planted on the ground.

There's a strain in your right leg.

After 15 to 30 seconds of holding, switch sides.

6. Wall-supported Quadriceps Stretch: Place your feet hip-width apart and face the wall.

Hold your right ankle with your right hand and feel the stretch at the front of your thigh as you push your right heel towards your buttocks, using the wall for support.

After 15 to 30 seconds of holding, switch sides.

7. Wall Ankle Stretch: Sit with your legs straight out in front of you and your back against the wall.

Place the top of your flexed right foot against the wall.

Feel the strain in your ankle as you gently press your toes on the wall.

After 15 to 30 seconds of holding, switch sides.

Some Advice on Moderate Wall-Based Stretches:

Utilize the Wall as Support:

For certain stretches, the wall offers support and stability.

Mild Motions:

To prevent tension, move slowly and gently through each stretch.

Inhaling:

Take regular, deep breaths while performing each stretch.

Breathe in from your nose, out through your mouth.

Comfortable Scope:

Only extend until you feel tension, not pain.
Reduce the intensity of the stretch if it hurts.
Continuity:

Incorporate these stretches into your everyday regimen to preserve suppleness and alleviate stress.
Adjust as Necessary:

Adapt the stretches to your level of comfort and any physical restrictions.
Remain Aware:

Take note of your body's needs and modify the stretches accordingly.
Speak with a healthcare provider if you have any concerns.
For those seeking a gentle and supportive way to stretch, try these wall-based stretches. They can be done on a regular basis to improve relaxation, ease tension, and increase flexibility. Always modify the stretches to suit your own requirements and comfort level, and get medical advice if you have any questions or concerns about your health.

Deep Breathing Exercises

Exercises involving deep breathing can be beneficial for relieving stress, improving general wellbeing, and relaxing. Including deep breathing exercises in your regimen can assist improve focus, induce awareness, and soothe the nervous system. You can attempt the following deep breathing exercises:

1. Diaphragmatic Breathing, often known as abdominal breathing: Take a comfortable seat or lie down.
Grasp your abdomen with one hand and your chest with the other.
Breathe deeply through your nose, letting your stomach grow. Sensate the diaphragm descend.
Breathe out slowly from your lips, allowing your stomach to contract.
Repeat a few times, paying attention to the rise and fall of your abdomen.
2. Box breathing, also known as square breathing: Take a comfortable seat and inhale for four counts via your nose.
For four counts, hold your breath.
Breathe out slowly through your mouth for four counts.
Take a four-count pause and hold your breath.

Continue this cycle for a few rounds, progressively raising the count if you feel comfortable doing so.

3. 4-7-8 Breathing (Relaxing Breath): Find a comfortable spot to sit or lie down.

Silently inhale through your nostrils and count to four in your head.

For seven counts, hold your breath.

Make a whooshing sound and exhale fully through your mouth to the count of eight.

Continue in this manner for multiple breaths.

4. Switching Nostril Breathing (Nadi Shodhana): Take a comfortable seat and maintain a straight spine.

Close your right nostril with your thumb, then take a breath through your left.

Using your right ring finger to close your left nostril, open your right nose, and let out a breath.

Breathe in using your right nostril.

Shut your right nose, open your left, and let out a breath.

Repeat a few times, paying attention to the flow of your breaths.

5. Mindful Breathing: Select a peaceful area and take a comfortable seat.

Shut your eyes and focus on your breathing. Take a slow, deep breath and pay attention to how it feels entering your body.

Feel the tension melting as you fully exhale.

Keep your attention on each breath and let go of any outside distractions.
If your thoughts stray, practice awareness by gently bringing them back to the breath.
Guidelines for Deep Breathing Exercises: Regular Practice

Even if you just have a little window of time each day, set aside time specifically for deep breathing exercises.
A cozy setting

Select a peaceful, comfortable area where you can concentrate without interruptions.
Regularity is Essential:

Duration is not as crucial as consistency. Frequent short sessions can be more productive than long ones that happen once in a while.
Position:

For best breathing, sit or lie down in a comfortable position with a straight spine.
Conscious Awareness:

Pay attention to your breath. If your thoughts stray, softly return them to the breath.
Recognize Your Needs:

Select a breathing exercise that you find relaxing and modify the methods to fit your comfort level. Talking with:

Before beginning deep breathing exercises, speak with a healthcare provider if you have any respiratory or other health issues.

There are several advantages to incorporating deep breathing into your routine for both your physical and emotional health. Try out several methods until you find ones that work for you, and incorporate deep breathing into your daily self-care regimen.

Mindful Relaxation Techniques

It can be beneficial to use mindful relaxation techniques to lower stress, foster calmness, and improve general wellbeing. By paying attention to the current moment without passing judgment, you can incorporate mindfulness into your daily practice. You can experiment with the following several mindful relaxation techniques:

1. Body Scan Meditation: Take a seat or lie down in a comfortable posture.

Shut your eyes and concentrate on your breathing.

Mentally begin to scan your body, working your way up from your toes.

Take note of any feelings, tense spots, or calm spots.

Breathe into any tense spots and give them permission to relax.

2. Mindful Breathing: Take a comfortable seat and concentrate on your inhalation.

As you count to four, carefully inhale through your nose.

Breathe out from your mouth while counting to six.

Take note of how your breath feels as it enters and exits your body.

Bring your thoughts back to the breath slowly if they stray.

3. Guided Imagery: Locate a peaceful area where you can lie down or sit.

Shut your eyes and picture a serene location, like a meadow, forest, or beach.

During the images, use all of your senses. What do you hear, see, smell, and feel?

Permit yourself to get carried away by the soothing feelings of the imagined scene.

4. Practice Loving-Kindness Meditation: Close your eyes while sitting comfortably.

Love and kindness should be directed first towards yourself.

Feel the same way for friends, family, and eventually all living things.

Say things like "May I/you be happy, may I/you be healthy, may I/you be safe, may I/you be at ease."

5. Mindful Walking: Pick a peaceful area to stroll, either inside or outside.

Take your time, move gently, and focus on each step while you walk.

Take note of how your feet are raising, moving, and touching the ground.

Remain mindful and observe your environment objectively.

6. Progressive Muscle Relaxation (PMR): Locate a calm, cozy area in which to sit or lay.

Start with your toes, tensing and then relaxing the muscles for a little while.

As you increase gradually, tense and release each muscle group.

Observe how stress and relaxation feel in your body.

7. Mindful Eating: Select a tiny serving of food, such as a slice of fruit or a raisin.

With curiosity, examine the food, taking note of its color, texture, and shape.

Take a whiff of its perfume and note any taste sensations.

Taste it slowly, concentrating on the textures and flavors.

Observe every chew and the swallowing experience.

Suggestions for Intentional Calm:

Begin Little:

Start off with brief sessions and then increase the length as you get more accustomed to the routines.

Continuity:

For optimal effects, integrate awareness into your everyday activities.

Nonjudgmental Consciousness:

Approach every technique with an accepting and non-critical attitude. Embrace whatever comes up without passing judgment.

Try this:

Investigate many methods to determine which one most appeals to you.

Employ Resources:

If you struggle to practice mindfulness on your own, think about using apps or guided meditations.

Give it a Personal Touch:

Tailor mindfulness exercises to your requirements and inclinations.
Have patience:

Being mindful is a talent that comes with practice. Have patience with yourself while you develop these habits.
Seek Advice:

If you're just starting out with mindfulness, think about going to classes or getting advice from seasoned practitioners.
Techniques for mindful relaxation can be effective tools for stress management and wellbeing promotion. Including these routines in your everyday life will help you approach obstacles and events with greater awareness and balance.

28 Days Workout Planners

Weekly Workout Planner

MONDAY	TUESDAY	WEDNESDAY

THURSDAY	FRIDAY	SATURDAY

NOTES

Weekly Workout Planner

MONDAY

TUESDAY

WEDNESDAY

THURSDAY

FRIDAY

SATURDAY

NOTES

Weekly Workout Planner

MONDAY

TUESDAY

WEDNESDAY

THURSDAY

FRIDAY

SATURDAY

NOTES

Weekly Workout Planner

MONDAY

TUESDAY

WEDNESDAY

THURSDAY

FRIDAY

SATURDAY

NOTES